UNDERSTANDING VOLUMETRICS

A COMPREHENSIVE GUIDE TO HEALTHY EATING

CYRIL LAKES

Contents

CHAPTER ONE

INTRODUCTION

A dietary strategy known as volumetrics emphasizes eating foods with a low energy density, or fewer calories per gram. Dr. Barbara Rolls, a nutrition researcher, created the Volumetrics diet plan, which stresses consuming foods rich in volume but low in calories, like fruits, vegetables, broth-based soups, and lean proteins, to help people feel full and content in less time.

Regardless of the food's calorie content, humans typically eat a same volume or weight of food each day, which is the foundation of the volumetrics theory. People can eat more food in greater portions without ingesting too many calories by selecting meals with high fiber, water, or air content. This can help you lose weight or keep it off without making you feel hungry or deprived.

In contrast to other trendy eating plans that emphasize limiting or doing away with specific food groups, Volumetrics encourages a flexible and well-rounded eating style. It promotes eating more nutrient-dense meals first while allowing for infrequent, moderation-based pleasures.

This introduction to Volumetrics will cover the fundamental ideas behind the method, its advantages, and how to incorporate it into a healthy lifestyle for long-term weight loss and general wellbeing.

An Overview of Volumetric Measurements

Dr. Barbara Rolls, a nutrition specialist, created the volumetrics diet plan, which emphasizes eating foods low in energy density to help control weight and improve general health. The fundamental tenet of volumetrics is that people can choose foods with a high volume but low calorie content to feel full and satisfied while consuming less calories.

The foundation of volumetrics is the idea of energy density. Calorie density is the quantity of calories in a specific amount of food by weight or volume. meals that are high in energy density deliver more calories per gram than meals that are low in energy density.

Low-energy-density meals including fruits, vegetables, broth-based soups, whole grains, and lean proteins are recommended to be consumed by volumetrics. These foods provide volume to the diet without dramatically raising calorie consumption since they are usually high in water, fiber, or air content. People who choose low-energy-density foods are able to consume less calories while yet feeling satisfied and eating greater servings.

On the other hand, the Volumetrics approach advocates consuming foods high in energy density—like fried foods, processed snacks, sugary drinks, and fatty meats—in moderation or in little amounts. Due to their high calorie content, these meals may cause weight gain if overindulged.

The Volumetrics method emphasizes nutrient-dense foods and allows for occasional indulgences while encouraging a flexible and balanced diet. It encourages people to make healthier eating choices by paying attention to the energy density of foods rather than relying on rigorous calorie tracking or portion management.

People can enhance overall nutritional quality, accomplish sustained weight loss or maintenance, and lower their chance of developing chronic diseases linked to obesity by adhering to the principles of volumetrics.

Furthermore, emphasizing hearty, nutrient-dense foods can enhance sustained adherence to good eating practices by preventing hunger and promoting fullness.

All things considered, Volumetrics provides a workable and empirically based strategy for reaching and keeping a healthy weight while taking pleasure in a filling and nourishing meal.

The history and development of the volumetrics method

Dr. Barbara Rolls, a nutrition researcher and professor of nutritional sciences at The Pennsylvania State University, created the volumetrics eating method. Dr. Rolls has dedicated decades of research to the scientific study of hunger, fullness, and the regulation of food intake. Specifically, he has examined the effects of food volume and calorie density on eating patterns and weight control.

Dr. Rolls' curiosity about the reasons behind people's propensity to overeat and put on weight—even when they are consuming foods labeled as "low-fat" or "diet" options—led to the creation of Volumetrics. Regardless of the food's calorie composition, Dr. Rolls' research revealed that the amount ingested is a significant factor in determining feelings of pleasure and fullness.

Early studies by Dr. Rolls showed that foods with a lower energy density and larger volume, such veggies, fruits, and broth-based soups, can more effectively fill the stomach and cause the brain to send satiety signals, which can reduce overall calorie consumption. On the other hand, foods with a high energy density, such sweets, fried foods, and fatty snacks, tend to be less satisfying and can cause overindulgence and weight gain.

Dr. Rolls created the Volumetrics approach in response to these findings, emphasizing the intake of low-energy-density meals to assist people in controlling their weight and enhancing the quality of their diet overall. The Volumetrics strategy promotes reducing the consumption of calorie-dense foods and giving priority to foods rich in volume but low in calories, such as fruits, vegetables, whole grains, and lean proteins.

Dr. Rolls and her research team have carried out a great deal of research over the years, including several studies and clinical trials, to find out more about how well the Volumetrics approach works for managing weight and general health. In comparison to those on other diets, their research continuously demonstrates that people who adhere to the principles of volumetrics tend to consume less calories, feel more satisfied and full, and achieve sustained weight loss or weight maintenance.

The Volumetrics method is now well known as a realistic and scientifically supported way to reach and maintain a healthy weight while having a tasty and nourishing food. The innovative research conducted by Dr. Rolls has greatly advanced our knowledge of eating behavior and shaped public health guidelines aimed at encouraging better eating practices.

An explanation of the philosophy and guiding ideas

The theory and fundamentals of the Volumetrics eating method are based on the science of satiety, appetite control, and weight management. The following explains the main ideas and mindset that underpin volumetrics:

Emphasis on Energy Density: The main idea behind volumetrics is to give preference to foods with low energy densities, or fewer calories per gram. These foods, which add volume to the diet without dramatically boosting calorie consumption, include fruits, vegetables, whole grains, broth-based soups, and lean proteins. They are also high in water, fiber, or air content. People can eat larger portions and feel fuller while yet consuming fewer calories overall by concentrating on foods with low energy density.

Eat More, Weigh Less: Volumetrics refutes the idea that severe restriction or portion control are necessary for losing weight. Rather, it places emphasis on consuming foods that are bigger in volume but lower in calories, enabling people to consume filling quantities without going over their daily calorie intake limit. People can lose weight or maintain their current weight by consuming a diet high in nutrients and low in energy density without experiencing hunger pangs or deprivation.

Balance and Moderation: Although volumetrics promotes the consumption of items low in energy density, it also stresses moderation and balance in dietary selections. The Volumetrics strategy does not exclude any foods, although it does advise consuming calorie-dense items like sweets, fried dishes, and fatty snacks in moderation. The secret is to balance your consumption of calories while consuming meals that are high in energy density and rich in nutrients yet low in density.

Volumetrics acknowledges the role that fullness and satisfaction play in encouraging sustained adherence to a healthy diet over the long term.

People are less likely to feel hungry or have cravings when they choose foods that are filling and satisfying, which lowers the chance of overindulging and improves adherence to dietary guidelines. Foods rich in protein, fiber, and water are especially good for fostering sensations of pleasure and fullness.

Integrating Dietary Principles with a Healthy Lifestyle: Volumetrics places a strong emphasis on the integration of dietary principles with a healthy lifestyle that include regular physical activity, stress reduction, and enough sleep. Along with other lifestyle choices, eating a balanced and sustainable diet helps long-term weight control success and enhances general health and well-being.

CHAPTER TWO

Overall, volumetrics is a flexible and sustainable eating strategy that emphasizes nutrient-dense, low-energy foods while allowing for enjoyment and satisfaction. It is based on scientific facts and practical considerations. People can improve their overall dietary quality and well-being and reach their weight reduction or weight maintenance goals by adhering to the fundamental principles of volumetrics.

Volumetrics: The Science Behind It

Dr. Barbara Rolls and her colleagues' multi-decade research on the connections between food volume, energy density, satiety, and weight control forms the foundation of Volumetrics science. The following summarizes the main scientific ideas that support the Volumetrics method:

Energy Density: The amount of calories in a specific amount of food by weight or volume is referred to as energy density. meals that are high in energy density deliver more calories per gram than meals that are low in energy density. According to Dr. Rolls' research, regardless of the food's calorie composition, people typically eat a similar volume or weight of food each day. People can consume fewer calories overall by eating greater quantities of foods with low energy density.

Foods with a higher volume and lower energy density have the ability to fill the stomach and cause satiety signals to be sent to the brain, as evidenced by Dr. Rolls' studies. These foods, which are usually high in fiber, water, or air content, encourage feelings of pleasure and fullness, which lowers the risk of overindulging. People can more successfully control their food intake and weight by giving priority to foods that increase fullness.

Portion Size and Calorie Intake: Research indicates that people typically consume a same amount of food regardless of how many calories it contains every day. People can eat more food without substantially increasing their calorie consumption if they choose meals with a low energy density. This enables weight loss or weight maintenance objectives to be met while also allowing for increased meal satisfaction and enjoyment.

Nutrient Density: Volumetrics emphasizes the importance of nutrient density in food choices, but it also concentrates on energy density. Foods high in nutrients offer vital vitamins, minerals, and other nutrients that promote general health and wellbeing. People can obtain the nutrients they need while controlling their weight by giving priority to foods that are high in nutrients and low in energy density.

Long-Term Sustainability: The Volumetrics approach's emphasis on adherence and long-term sustainability is one of its main advantages. Volumetrics encourages a long-term, sustainable, and balanced approach to eating by promoting the consumption of nutrient-dense, enjoyable meals in sensible portions. People are more likely to maintain a healthy lifestyle and reach their weight loss or weight management objectives as a result.

All things considered, the study of volumetrics offers a strong basis for comprehending how meal volume, energy density, and nutrient density affect eating patterns, feelings of fullness, and the regulation of body weight. By putting these guidelines into practice, people can enjoy wholesome, delicious meals and make educated food choices that promote their health and wellbeing.

Recognizing the Volumetrics Dietary Plan

The goal of the Volumetrics eating plan is to help people control their weight and enhance the overall quality of their diet by emphasizing low-energy density foods. This is an explanation of the Volumetrics eating plan's operation:

Stress on Low-Energy-Density Foods: Eating foods with a low energy density is the foundation of the Volumetrics diet plan. Compared to foods with a greater energy density, these items—which include fruits, vegetables, whole grains, broth-based soups, and lean proteins—provide less calories per gram. People can consume higher quantities of low-energy-density meals and still consume less calories overall by doing so.

Fill Up on Fruits and Vegetables: since of their high water and fiber content, fruits and vegetables are essential parts of the Volumetrics eating plan since they increase meal volume without dramatically raising calorie intake. These meals should be the main course of every meal and should be eaten in large quantities.

Incorporate Lean Proteins and entire Grains: The Volumetrics eating plan places a strong emphasis on entire grains like brown rice, quinoa, and barley as well as lean proteins like chicken, fish, beans, and tofu. These foods contribute vital nutrients and aid in satiety, increasing the satisfaction and fillingness of meals.

Limit High-Energy-Density Foods: The Volumetrics eating plan does not forbid any foods, but it does advise consuming higher-energy-density items including processed foods, sweets, fried foods, and fatty snacks in moderation. Due to their high calorie content, these meals may cause weight gain if overindulged.

Eat Mindfully: The Volumetrics eating plan promotes mindful eating, which is eating deliberately, savoring each meal, and paying attention to indications of hunger and fullness. It is possible for people to better control their food intake and prevent overeating by paying attention to portion sizes and listening to their bodies.

Keep Yourself Hydrated: Another key component of the Volumetrics eating plan is drinking lots of water and other calorie-free liquids. Water facilitates feelings of fullness and helps the stomach fill up, which makes it simpler to watch portion sizes and cut back on calories.

Include Physical Activity: As part of a healthy lifestyle, frequent physical activity is suggested even though the Volumetrics eating plan largely focuses on food choices. Engaging in physical activity promotes calorie burning, muscle growth, and general health and wellbeing.

All things considered, the Volumetrics eating plan provides a durable and adaptable method of maintaining a healthy weight. People can enjoy pleasant and nutritious meals while achieving their weight loss or weight management goals by emphasizing nutrient-dense, low-energy-density foods and paying attention to portion sizes.

The Volumetrics Approach's advantages

The Volumetrics method has various advantages for people who want to control their weight and enhance their general health:

Satiety and Fullness: The Volumetrics approach encourages feelings of fullness and satisfaction by emphasizing low-energy-density foods that are high in volume, fiber, and water content. This can promote weight management by assisting people in managing their appetite, lowering desires for food, and preventing overindulging.

Increased Nutrient Intake: The Volumetrics strategy makes sure that people obtain the vital vitamins, minerals, and other nutrients they need for optimum health by placing an emphasis on nutrient-dense meals like fruits, vegetables, lean proteins, and whole grains. People can enhance the overall quality of their diet and meet their nutritional requirements by giving priority to certain foods.

Sustainable Weight Loss: The Volumetrics approach enables people to eat satisfying portions of nutrient-rich foods without feeling restricted, in contrast to many fad diets that rely on stringent calorie tracking or food limitations. This facilitates long-term adherence to the eating plan, which results in weight loss and maintenance that is sustainable.

Flexibility and diversity: People can design meals that fit their tastes and lifestyles thanks to the Volumetrics approach's flexibility and diversity of food options. With so many options for low-energy-density foods, people can still meet their dietary requirements and enjoy a variety of tasty meals.

Better Eating Habits: By using the Volumetrics technique, people are encouraged to choose whole, minimally processed foods over calorie-dense, nutrient-poor ones. This can eventually result in better eating habits, a decrease in the consumption of bad foods, and an increased appreciation for filling, healthful meals.

Reduced Risk of Chronic Disease: Obesity, type 2 diabetes, heart disease, and some malignancies can all be prevented by according to the Volumetrics approach's guiding principles, which place an emphasis on eating fruits, vegetables, whole grains, and lean proteins. Volumetrics enhances general health and well-being by encouraging a diet that is nutrient-rich and well-balanced.

Improved Quality of Life: Using the Volumetrics technique to reach and maintain a healthy weight can result in better physical and mental health as well as more energy and a stronger sense of overall wellbeing. Volumetrics helps people live better lives and confidently pursue their personal and professional objectives by promoting general health and energy.

All things considered, the Volumetrics method provides a workable and empirically based plan for reaching and keeping a healthy weight while savoring filling and nourishing meals. With its emphasis on mindful eating, portion control, and low-energy-density meals, Volumetrics enables people to transform their eating behaviors for the better and enhance their long-term health and well-being.

Applying Volumetric Measurements

Applying Volumetrics entails integrating its tenets into your regular dietary routine. Here's how to put the Volumetrics method into practice:

Put Low-Energy-Density meals First: Stuff your plate full of low-energy-density meals like fruits, vegetables, nutritious grains, soups with broth, and lean meats. These foods satisfy your hunger and give you volume without adding too many calories.

Start with Soup or Salad: To start meals, have a big salad full of bright vegetables and leafy greens, or a soup with a broth basis. This lowers the total number of calories consumed during the meal by filling you full with high-volume, low-calorie items.

Increase the Volume of veggies in Your Meals: When making stir-fries, pasta meals, or casseroles, make sure to include a good amount of veggies. Vegetables reduce the amount of calories in meals while increasing volume, fiber, and minerals.

Select Whole Grains: Refined grains should be avoided in favor of whole grains such brown rice, quinoa, barley, and whole wheat bread. Because whole grains have more minerals and fiber per calorie, they are more satiating.

Lean Protein Sources: Include lean protein sources in your meals, such as fish, chicken, beans, lentils, tofu, and low-fat dairy. Overall satiety is increased by protein because it maintains muscular health and helps to create sensations of fullness.

Restrict High-Energy-Density items: Although there are no items that are off-limits, when consuming foods high in energy density, like sweets, fried foods, and fatty snacks, pay attention to portion sizes and frequency. Eat these meals in moderation as special occasions only, not as mainstays of your diet.

Practice Portion Control: Be mindful of serving sizes and take suitable portions for your level of hunger and satiety. Reduce the size of your dishes and bowls to help you eat less and not overindulge.

Keep Yourself Hydrated: A lot of water should be consumed throughout the day because often dehydration is confused with hunger. To help you feel fuller and stay hydrated, choose calorie-free drinks like sparkling water, herbal tea, or water.

Eat mindfully by taking your time, enjoying every bite, and being aware of your body's signals of hunger and fullness. Eat without interruptions from electronics or television to savor your meal to the fullest and avoid thoughtless overeating.

Include Physical Activity: To enhance general health and weight management, combine the Volumetrics strategy with frequent physical activity. Aim for two or more days of muscle-strengthening exercises each week in addition to at least 150 minutes of moderate-intensity activity or 75 minutes of vigorous-intensity exercise per week.

You may successfully apply the principles of Volumetrics to your daily life and reap the benefits of a satisfying, nutrient-dense diet that promotes weight management and overall well-being by putting these tactics into practice and gradually altering your eating habits.

Integrating Physical Activity and Exercise

Including physical activity and exercise in your routine is a key element of the Volumetrics method to managing your weight and your general health. Here's how to incorporate physical activity into your daily routine:

Select Pleasurable Activities: Opt for pursuits that you sincerely find enjoyable and eager to engage in. Finding engaging and fun activities to engage in, whether it be walking, swimming, cycling, dancing, yoga, or sports, will help you stay motivated and dedicated to regular exercise.

Establish Achievable Goals: Whether it's stepping up your daily activity, deciding on a weekly exercise schedule, or aiming for particular fitness benchmarks, set realistic goals for yourself. As you advance, progressively raise the duration or intensity of your workouts from small, realistic targets.

Make It a Habit: Include regular workouts in your weekly schedule and regard them as non-negotiable appointments. To get the most out of fitness, you should try to work out most days of the week. Consistency is essential.

Add Variety: To keep things fresh and avoid monotony, mix up your routine by including a range of exercise styles. A well-rounded fitness program makes sure you're working diverse muscle groups and getting the benefits of cardio, weight training, flexibility, and balancing activities.

Be Active Throughout the Day: Even when you're not doing structured exercise sessions, try to find ways to fit in some physical activity each day. When feasible, avoid driving and opt for walking or biking instead of taking the elevator. Additionally, try to intersperse brief exercise breaks between extended periods of sitting.

CHAPTER THREE

Listen to Your Body: During and after exercise, pay attention to how your body feels. Then, modify the intensity or length of your workout as necessary. It's crucial to push oneself, but not to the point of fatigue or harm. Respect your body's demands and allow yourself to recuperate when needed.

Have Reasonable Expectations: Remind yourself that growth takes time and exercise patience with yourself. When you encounter obstacles or roadblocks along the route, don't give up. No matter how tiny your accomplishments may be, acknowledge them and concentrate on the constructive adjustments you're creating to enhance your wellbeing.

Seek Support and Accountability: To get accountability, support, and inspiration, find a workout partner, enroll in a fitness class, or work with a personal trainer. It might be more fun and keep you motivated to reach your objectives if you have someone to share your fitness journey with.

You can obtain a balanced and sustainable approach to managing your weight and general health by implementing the concepts of the Volumetrics eating plan together with frequent exercise and physical activity into your lifestyle. It's important to prioritize enjoyable hobbies, develop reasonable goals, and incorporate physical activity into your daily routine.

Testimonials and Success Stories

Testimonials and success stories from people who have used the Volumetrics technique can serve as a source of motivation and inspiration for those who want to control their weight and improve their health. Here are few instances:

Sarah's Weight Loss Journey: Sarah battled for years to control her weight, going through a number of diets and feeling famished and hungry all the time. She made the decision to give the Volumetrics approach a shot after learning about it. Sarah discovered that she could have fulfilling meals and still lose weight by concentrating on hearty, low-energy-density foods and controlling her portion sizes. Sarah had a thirty-pound weight loss and an increase in energy and confidence over the course of six months. She believes that the Volumetrics method has transformed her connection with food and enabled her to lose weight in a way that will last.

John's Health Transformation: After receiving a diagnosis of prediabetes and high cholesterol, John realized he needed to drastically alter his food and way of life in order to become better. He discovered about the Volumetrics approach and made the decision to give it a try after speaking with a nutritionist. John was able to lower his blood sugar, normalize his cholesterol, and shed extra weight by limiting higher-energy-density foods and placing an emphasis on fruits, vegetables, lean proteins, and whole grains. He is thankful for Volumetrics' beneficial influence on his health and wellbeing, as he feels better than ever.

Emily's Path to Better Eating Habits: For years, Emily battled emotional eating and yo-yo dieting, feeling caught in a vicious cycle of guilt-ridden binge eating. She changed her perspective on her relationship with food after learning about the Volumetrics principles. Emily realized that she could overcome her bad eating habits and create a more balanced eating routine by concentrating on nutrient-dense, low-energy-density foods and engaging in mindful eating. She has learnt to enjoy meals guilt-free and without any restrictions, and she no longer thinks that food controls her. Emily's experience with Volumetrics has had a profoundly positive emotional and physical impact.

These endorsements and success stories show how the Volumetrics method can improve one's general health, well-being, and ability to control weight. Healthy eating practices and a focus on nutrient-dense, low-energy meals can help people reach their weight loss and health objectives in a fun and sustainable way.

Summary

To sum up, the Volumetrics eating method provides a realistic, scientifically supported means of controlling weight, enhancing general health, and improving overall well-being. People can enjoy fulfilling meals while still reaching their weight reduction or weight maintenance goals by emphasizing low-energy-density foods, giving nutrient-rich options priority, and exercising portion control.

Volumetrics emphasizes the significance of eating a balanced and sustainable diet that emphasizes whole grains, fruits, vegetables, lean proteins, and low-fat foods while limiting higher-energy-density items. This strategy helps people maintain their ideal weight while simultaneously lowering their chance of developing chronic illnesses, improving the quality of their diet, and developing long-term healthy eating habits.

Testimonials and success stories from people who have adopted the Volumetrics approach demonstrate how well it works to change people's lives and give them the confidence to take charge of their health. The advantages of Volumetrics go far beyond the number on the scale, whether it's conquering obstacles related to managing weight, enhancing metabolic health markers, or cultivating a better connection with food.

The Volumetrics strategy can be made even more effective by adding regular exercise, drinking enough of water, eating mindfully, and asking for help when needed. People can see long-lasting gains in their vitality, health, and general quality of life by gradually altering their dietary and lifestyle choices.

All things considered, the Volumetrics method provides a workable, adaptable, and pleasurable means of attaining long-term weight loss, encouraging ideal health, and cultivating a constructive rapport with food. People can start on a path to a better, happier, and more fulfilled life by accepting its ideas and making empowered decisions.

THE END